HOW CAN I GET PREGNANT

NATURALLY?

KIBOKO FRANÇOISE MACHOZI

www.savelife.co.za

CONTENTS

INTRODUCTION

While practicing back home in the Democratic Republic of Congo, I had several patients consult me about infertility problems. Before I referred them to a gynecologist, I used to ask some questions and give them known guidelines, which, in some cases, worked very well—in less than a year, some of the ladies were pregnant.
This motivated me to write this book because sometimes the problem is not as serious as we think, and a simple guideline may be the solution.

The process of becoming pregnant is natural. A couple may not need any extra effort for a woman to get pregnant, but it can happen that a woman may struggle to get pregnant, although she is healthy and able to conceive. In such a case, the woman needs to know about her body and how it works.

It can happen that a couple wanting to bear a child is having sex at the wrong time. This is common when the two are working different shifts or when one or both of them are traveling regularly.

For a woman to conceive, she must have sexual intercourse during or around her ovulation. Only sexual intercourse done during or around ovulation will be fruitful, even though one's state of mind has a role to play in getting pregnant (and a deep desire to conceive may actually delay the process).

1. ANATOMY OF A FEMALE REPRODUCTIVE SYSTEM

The female reproductive system is subdivided into two different parts: the internal and the external part (or vulva).

1. 1. INTERNAL FEMALE REPRODUCTIVE SYSTEM

1. UTERUS

The uterus is a median, pear-shaped, hollow, muscular, and elastic organ in which the fertilized ovum becomes an embryo, a fetus, and, later, a baby. It is situated in the pelvis between the bladder at the front and the rectum at the back side.

It is composed of two parts: the body (the upper part) and the cervix (lower part), which opens into the vagina below and into the uterine cavity above.

The uterus has three layers:

- the endometrium or inner layer of the uterus cavity, on which a fertilized ovum fixes itself

(NB: Damage to the endometrium may cause adhesion and fibrosis, which are not favorable for the fixation of a fertilized ovum.)

- the myometrium or uterus muscles
- the perimetrium or uterus envelope

The uterus weighs between fifty and seventy grams. It measures approximately seven and half centimeters in length.[1]

2. VAGINA

The vagina is an elastic and muscular canal going from the lower part of the uterus (cervix) to the vulva. It measures approximately nine centimeters in length and six to seven and half centimeters in diameter.

Its roles consist of allowing intercourse, the passage of sperm to the uterus, the passage of menstruations to the vulva, and the passage of a child during birth.

The vagina allows the examination of the uterine cervix. It also allows different maneuvers to be performed in the uterus.

Bartholin glands or greater vestibular glands are two mucoid-secreting glands located in the lower part of the vagina, one at the left side and the other at the right. These glands produce a mucoid substance, which makes the vagina smooth and wet to avoid dryness and irritation.[ii]

3. FALLOPIAN TUBES

Fallopian tubes are two canals situated on both the left and the right sides of the upper lateral part of the uterus body. Each fallopian tube measures seven to fourteen centimeters in length. Fallopian tubes connect the uterus to the ovaries, allowing the passage of both spermatozoids from the uterus and ovum from the ovary to meet each other inside it. Fallopian tubes also allow the passage of a fertilized egg to the uterus.

Cilia and fluids found inside the fallopian tubes allow an ovum and a fertilized egg to move smoothly toward the uterus.

A fallopian tube has four parts:

- isthmus which is a narrower part that links to the cavity of the uterus
- ampulla (the portion where a spermatozoid meets an ovum)
- infundibulum which is the third part of a Fallopian tube that is situated between the ampoulla and the fimbria
- fimbria which is the last part of the fallopian tube in the direction of the ovary and which captures the egg once it is delivered by the ovary.

A fertilized egg takes seven days (from the ampulla) before it reaches the uterus.

A fallopian tube has three layers:

- Mucosa is the internal layer, which has ciliated cells.
- Muscularis (muscle) is the middle layer of a fallopian tube, which has nerves and allows motion.
- Serosa is the external layer or envelope of a fallopian tube.[iii]

4. OVARIES

Ovaries are oval organs situated at the end of each fallopian tube. They deliver an ovum once a month and produce hormones.[iv]

1. 2. THE EXTERNAL FEMALE REPRODUCTIVE SYSTEM

1. Labium majus are two lateral structures that cover and protect the external female reproductive system from germs.
They have glands that produce sweat and oil to protect the external female reproductive system from dryness and irritation.

2. Labium minus are folds of mucous membrane located at the left and right sides of the vaginal entrance. They have their origins in the lower part of the clitoris. They cover and protect the vaginal entrance from germs.

3. The clitoris is an erectile organ found in the anterior part of the vulva.

4. The vaginal orifice is a small hole situated in the middle posterior part of the vulva under the

two labium minus, between the orifices of both the urethra and the anus at the back side.[v]

2. FEMALE HORMONES

Hormones are chemical substances produced by glands. They move inside the body through the bloodstream and regulate the functions of others organs. Hormones work like messengers between different organs inside a human body.

Sex glands produce hormones during fetal development, but they become inactive during childhood.

At birth, a baby girl has 450,000 eggs in her ovaries. Each of them is found in an envelope called a follicle. At puberty, a teenager's body starts to produce hormones that mature her eggs. Female hormones are produced by ovaries. They produce estrogen, progesterone, and much more.

In this section we will focus on estrogen and progesterone. Estrogen builds up the uterine lining, thickens the vaginal lining, stimulates the breast tissue, promotes the building of bones, and protects the cardiovascular system.[vi]

Progesterone prepares the uterine lining to bear the fertilized ovum, increases sexual desire, increases energy, and develops muscles.

3. MENSTRUAL CYCLE

The hypothalamus is a gland in a human being's brain controlling the menstrual cycle. It releases a chemical called "follicles stimulating hormones regulating factor," or FSH-RF, to give information to the pituitary (the second gland in the brain), so it may release FSH in the blood stream. FSH increases blood supply in ovaries and promotes the maturation of follicles in the ovaries.

The maturing follicle releases another hormone called estrogen, which thickens the uterus lining and prepares it to bear a child. Also, it changes the appearance of the cervical mucus, which becomes slippery and transparent like a raw egg.

High levels of estrogen decrease the basal temperature (vaginal temperature) and stimulate the hypothalamus to produce another chemical called "leutenizing hormones regulating factor" (LH-RF), which makes the pituitary gland release the leutenizing hormone (LH). This hormone makes the most mature follicle burst and release the egg. This process is called ovulation.

Before ovulation, the blood supply in the ovaries increases; there is a contraction of ligaments, which allows the ovaries to be closer to the fallopian tubes and easily transfer the egg from the ovary to the fallopian tube once it is released.

The cervix releases stretchy, clear mucus, which allows the easy passage of spermatozoid to meet the egg inside the fallopian tube. Inside the fallopian tube, the egg movement is made possible by cilia.

From ovulation to menstruation, the follicle that released an ovum is called a corpus luteum or "yellow body" because of its color. This produces estrogen and a large amount of progesterone for the maintenance of the pregnancy. If there is no fertilization, the yellow body becomes white, and it is called corpus albicans.

Progesterone increases basal temperature; it makes the glands of the uterus lining produce mucous, which covers the internal part of the uterus (endometrium). If there is no fertilization, the uterus lining will be destroyed and convert into menstruations.[vii]

MENSTRUATION OR MENSES

This is a physiologic bloody discharge that comes from the uterus and occurs every month. It is a common process for women from puberty to menopause.

WHAT IS A MENSTRUAL CYCLE LENGTH

A menstrual cycle is a period that starts from the first day of your last menstruation period until the day of your next menstruation.

How do you know the length of your menstrual cycle?

To know the length of your cycle, you have to write down the first day of your menstruations, and, after six to twelve months, you calculate the number of days between two menstruation periods.

For example:

In January, you had your menstruation on the fourteenth.

In February, you had your menstruation on the seventeenth.

In March, you had your menstruation on the seventeenth.

In April, you had your menstruation on the sixteenth.

In May, you had your menstruation on the twentieth.

In June, you had your menstruation on the twenty-second.

In July, you had your menstruation on the twenty-first.

In August, you had your menstruation on the seventeenth.

In September, you had your menstruation on the fourteenth.

In October, you had your menstruation on the fourteenth.

In November, you had your menstruation on the fifteenth.

In December, you had your menstruation on the fourteenth.

From January to February, there were thirty-five days before you menstruated.

From February to March, there were twenty-nine days before you menstruated.

From March to April, there were thirty-one days before you menstruated.

From April to May, there were thirty-five days before you menstruated.

From May to June, there were thirty-four days before you menstruated.

From June to July, there were thirty days before you menstruated.

From July to August, there were twenty-eight days before you menstruated.

From August to September, there were twenty-nine days before you menstruated.

From September to October, there were thirty-one days before you menstruated.

From October to November, there were thirty-three days before you menstruated.

From November to December, there were thirty days before you menstruated.

Your longest cycle has thirty-five days, and your shortest cycle has twenty-eight days.

The average cycle =
$$\frac{\text{your longest cycle} + \text{your shortest cycle}}{2}$$

$$35+28=63/2=31.5=32$$

ESTIMATION OF THE DATE OF YOUR NEXT MENSTRUATIONS

To estimate the day of your next menstruation, you have to know the length of your cycle, and, from there, you count down on a calendar the average number of days of your cycle, starting from the first day of your last menstruation forward and find out the approximate day of your next menstruation.

For example:

You had your last menstruation on January 3rd. Your cycle has approximately thirty-two days. Your next menstruation will be around February 3rd.

OVULATION

Ovulation is the liberation of an ovum by an ovary. This occurs once during a menstrual cycle.

To estimate the day of your ovulation, you first have to estimate the date of your next menstruation; from there, on the calendar count backward fourteen days toward the last menstruation, and the fifteenth day is your estimated day of ovulation.

This is the right time to have sex or to avoid it, depending on whether or not you want to get pregnant.

Menstruations always happen fourteen days after ovulation.

NB: Actually, there are specific tests that help you find out exactly when you will be ovulating by checking the urine or the saliva. Those tests may predict your ovulation day up to seven days beforehand.

OVULATION SIGNS

- Increase in the amount and texture of cervical mucus

(It stretches and becomes slippery and clear like a raw egg because of the sharp rise in estrogen.)

- Discomfort in the lower part of the abdomen

(This pain is interpreted as tension caused by a follicle that is about to burst.)

- Slight bleeding in the middle of the cycle

- Change in position and firmness of the cervix

- Increased sexual desire

- Increased breast sensitivity

A sharp rise in body temperature is proof that you ovulated the day before.
After ovulation, the yellow body starts to produce progesterone, which increases the woman's body temperature.

A vaginal smear done during the first part of the cycle or follicular is clear, but the one done during the second part of the cycle or luteal is dirty.

An endometrium biopsy performed between the twenty-first and the twenty-fifth day of the cycle shows signs of ovulation.

A coelioscopy done in the middle of the cycle shows a mature follicle ready to rupture or already ruptured and transformed into a yellow body.

METHODS USED TO LOCATE THE APPROXIMATE TIME OF OVULATION

The menstrual cycle has two different phases:
The first phase or estrogenic phase—Its length may change due to different reasons, e.g., emotion, stress, diseases, weather, and much more.
The length of the second phase is constant and does not change due to any circumstance. The length is fourteen days. Once a woman ovulates, she has to count fourteen days before she will see her menstruations.

OVULATION CALENDAR

With this method, a woman will have to estimate the date of her next menstruation; from there, she will count backward fourteen days and can evaluate approximately the date on which she will be ovulating. To increase the chance of pregnancy, she should have sexual intercourse during this period.

EVALUATION OF CERVICAL MUCUS TEXTURE

To increase the likelihood of pregnancy, a woman will have to check and evaluate the texture, appearance, and color of her cervical mucus every morning, and she should have sexual intercourse once the texture of the cervical mucus increases and becomes slippery.

MEASURE OF BASAL TEMPERATURE

A woman wanting to conceive should check her vaginal temperature using a digital basal thermometer every morning. A day before ovulation, the temperature will decrease; once the temperature rises, the woman knows that she ovulated the day before.

URINE-BASED OVULATION TEST

This test is accurate and helps a woman know the exact day she ovulates.

FERTILITY MONITOR

This is a small machine that uses saliva to check the ovulation. This machine may predict ovulation up to seven days before by checking the level of progesterone, the level of estrogen, or both.

NB: An ovum may only live for twenty-four, hours while a spermatozoid may live up to five days. This means a woman may still become pregnant from sexual intercourse she had five days before ovulation and a day after ovulation.[viii]

4. CONDITIONS REQUIRED FOR A WOMAN TO CONCEIVE

For a woman to conceive, some conditions are required:
- The presence of a normal uterus, with at least one ovary and one unblocked tube
- Normal production of female hormones that induce ovulation
- Normal sexual intercourse during or around the ovulation day
- The presence of a healthy ovum and a healthy sperm
- A good state of mind

5. CONDITIONS REQUIRED FOR A MAN TO IMPREGNATE

For a man to impregnate a woman, there are four major conditions:

- His sexual glands must be able to produce enough spermatozoids that have a normal shape and mobility.

- A man must be able to release up to 20 million spermatozoids per cubic centimeter per ejaculation; among these, two hundred will reach the competitive stage, and only one will win the competition.
- The presence of a reproductive system that does not have abnormalities
- The ability to experience an erection and to perform normal sexual intercourse

6. DETERMINATION OF THE CHILD'S SEX

Men are responsible for the sex of the child as they release both chromosomes, X and Y. Women only have X chromosomes,
X chromosomes live longer but are slower.
Y chromosomes have a short lifetime but are quicker than the X ones.

A couple having sexual intercourse before ovulation has a high chance of conceiving a baby girl, and a couple having sexual intercourse after ovulation has a 100-percent chance of conceiving a baby boy.

NB: The problem with this is that despite all the modern tests detecting the ovulation day, it is still unpredictable.

7. STEPS TO HELP YOU CONCEIVE NATURALLY

When you are trying to conceive, you have to:
1. Consult your gynecologist together with your spouse and tell him/her that you are trying to bear a child.
a. He/she will proceed to give you a general checkup.
b. He/she will request some blood tests just to make sure that everything is fine since there are diseases that may delay conception, incrase your chances of bearing a child with abnormalities, or affect your pregnancy at its early stages or even later, and you may end up having a miscarriage, premature labor, or a stillborn; it may also happen that you conceive and deliver a baby who is also affected by the disease. In such a case, a doctor will provide you with a specific regimen to clear up the disease before you may conceive.

c. He/she will provide you with some immunizations to protect you and decrease the risk of developing some diseases that may affect your pregnancy.

d. He/she may also supply you with some medications if needed. Surgery may be required in the case of myoma, fibroid, and ovary cysts.

2. Have sexual intercourse around and on your ovulation day. Having sexual intercourse once per day is enough for you to conceive; you may even skip a day and perform only every two days.

3. Avoid stress and heightened emotions as these may delay conception or may lead to early miscarriage.

4. Do not be obsessed about getting pregnant because that may also delay conception.

BLOOD TESTS FOR WOMEN TRYING TO CONCEIVE

A woman trying to conceive will have to do some blood tests, which are as follows:

1. A hemoglobin blood test is done to make sure that the woman does not have anemia as it may compromise the life of the fetus.

2. An HIV test is done to diagnose HIV; if the woman tests positive, she must start her Anti Retroviral Treatment, and she will be advised to conceive only when the viral load becomes undetectable. This will protect her baby from the disease. If the diagnosis is made when the lady is already pregnant, she will have to start her ART as well. In both cases the gynecologist may stop the treatment after the woman has delivered depending on her CD4 count.

3. RPR (VDRL) is a blood test done to detect syphilis, which is a sexually transmissible disease. If the blood tests positive, the woman will take medications, along with her husband.

4. Serum Chlamydia: Test done to detect Clamidia, which is a sexually transmitted disease that may cause infertility (in both men and women), miscarriage, and ectopic pregnancy

(when a fertilized egg develops in a Fallopian tube).

5. German Measles or Rubella: a pregnant woman may pass the disease to the unborn child and cause congenital Rubella syndrome which is a condition characterized by deafness, sleepiness, irritability, skin rashes, cloudy cornea and may lead to Autism, growth retardation, learning disability, Schizophrenia, Diabetes and Glaucoma.

6. Hepatitis B is a blood test that detects antibodies to hepatitis B as the infection may lead to a premature labor, a lady may also deliver after nine months a mature baby but having a low birth weight.

7. Fasting glucose and fasting insulin to diagnose some metabolic disorders such as Diabetes Mellitus as this may delay a lady from conceiving, it may also lead to stillbirth, the lady may also deliver a living baby but having some abnormalities.

8. A blood group and rhesus factor is done to determine the nature of the blood of an individual, so, in a case of hemorrhage, a woman will receive the proper blood. If the Rhesus factor is negative, she will receive a vaccine

while she is pregnant and after delivery to protect her baby from death.

9. Hemoglobin electrophoresis is a blood test done to detect drepanocytosis and thalassemia, which are genetic diseases characterized by red blood cell abnormalities that may be transmitted to the baby.

10. Indirect coomb test is a test that detects antibodies that kill blood cells.

IMMUNIZATION FOR WOMEN TRYING TO CONCEIVE

A woman trying to conceive will receive some immunizations:

Flu vaccine
Yellow fever vaccine
Hepatitis B vaccine
Tetanus vaccine
Rubella vaccine
Diphteria and mumps vaccine

Some of these must be given before conception, not after, as they may lead to life-threatening diseases.

VITAMINS AND MINERAL SUPPLEMENTS

A woman trying to conceive must eat healthy foods. She must increase the intake of nuts, grains, fruits, and vegetables, as they are rich in vitamins and minerals that maintain the reproductive system. Food rich in good proteins, like chicken and eggs, fish rich in omega-3, and food rich in iron and selenium may regulate the secretion of hormones and boost fertility. She should take a supplement of folic acid from the time she decides to conceive; this will protect her baby from spina bifida (one of the congenital abnormalities of the spinal cord). A doctor may also prescribe other medications according to the blood test results.

She must exercise moderately on a regular basis to maintain her BMI, improve blood circulation, and eliminate toxins.[ix]

NB: Caffeine decreases fertility in both males and females.

FOODS TO AVOID WHILE TRYING TO CONCEIVE

Processed food
Raw fish and fish rich in mercury
Unpasteurized dairy products
Meat that contains nitrite
Undercooked food
Food that is not fresh or cleaned well
Sprouts
Coffee
Sugar-rich food
Fatty food
Alcohol
Tobacco[x]

8. PREGNANCY

Pregnancy is the state of a female after conception and until the termination of the gestation.[1]

Conception: fertilization of an ovum by a spermatozoid
Gestation: the fact of bearing a fertilized ovum

Having sex around or during ovulation does not guarantee pregnancy; many factors have to be considered before a woman can conceive (e.g., the receptivity of the uterus, her state of mind).

If it happens that you do not manage to conceive naturally after a year of trying, , you will have to consult your gynecologist again. (You do not need to change doctors for that because it is a process.)
The doctor will proceed to give you a fertility test (FSH, LH, thyroid function, free testosterone index, prolactine, progesterone, estradiol) on the second and third days of the

---

[1]*Stedman's Medical Dictionary for the Health Professions and Nursing*, illustrated 5th edition, page 1180

cycle with the purpose of evaluating if you are ovulating or not. If the test reveals that you are ovulating, the gynecologist will request other blood tests, such as a semen analysis (if the result is abnormal, a sperm antibodies test will be done).

At the same time, the gynecologist will attend to your husband/partner and give him the following tests: androgen profile, free testosterone index, prolactine, FSH/LH, spermogram.

If all the results are normal, the gynecologist will send you for a hystero salpingo gram, which is an X-ray done to visualize and to open blocked tubes. The process may be repeated up to three times, trying to open blocked tubes (if there are any).

A laparoscopy is recommended to investigate for endometriosis if the hystero salpingo gram does not reveal any abnormality.

If the fertility tests reveal that you do not ovulate, the doctor will prescribe some pills for you (e.g., Clomid) that will induce ovulation. He/she may repeat the process up to three times.

9. INFERTILITY

Infertility is the inability of a couple to conceive after one year of having regular (two to three times per week) and normal sexual intercourse. Eighty-five percent of couples manage to conceive after a year of having a normal and regular sex life, but 15 percent are still unable to bear a child after twelve months of normal and regular unprotected sexual intercourse.

Among them:
One-third involves male problems.
One-third involves female problems.
One-third does not have an apparent cause.

CAUSES OF MALE INFERTILITY

The causes of male infertility are as follow:

- An inadequate quantity of spermatozoids
For a male to impregnate, he must produce up to 20 million spermatozoids per cubic centimeter of semen since many of these will die before they reach the target (ovum), and only two hundred spermatozoids per squared millimeter

may reach the competitive stage, **but only one will win the race and fertilize an ovum.**

- An inadequate quality of spermatozoids

All spermatozoids are similar; they have an oval head and a long tail that allows motion. A male will experience infertility once the shape of his spermatozoids is different. For spermatozoids to reach and fertilize an ovum at the appropriate place, they must be mobile, as an ovum only lives for twenty-four hours.[xi]

CAUSES OF ALL THE SPERM PROBLEMS

The causes of spermatozoid problems are:
- Hormonal insufficiency
- Undescended testicles
- Abnormality or obstruction of testicular tubes

(This may be congenital or consecutive to some infections, previous surgery, or testicles trauma.)
- Cancer, chemotherapy, and radiotherapy
- Post-pubertal mumps
- Repeated sexually transmissible infections (gonorrhea, chlamydia)
- Genetic defects and genetic diseases

- Premature ejaculation
- Painful intercourse
- Erectile problems,
- Presence of anti-spermatozoid antibodies

(A male may produce antibodies against his spermatozoids; a woman may also produce antibodies against her husband's spermatozoids.)

- Poor nutrition and obesity
- Alcohol, tobacco, and drug consumption
- Repeated exposure to the heat (saunas), pesticides, and other chemicals
- Age
- Stress (as it interferes with hormones that produce spermatozoids)[xii]

ADVICE FOR A MAN WANTING TO BECOME A FATHER ONE DAY

All men wanting to be fathers one day have to:

- Avoid stress, as it interferes with hormones that produce spermatozoids.
- Lose weight, as obesity may lead to heart diseases and erectile problems; it reduces the number and the mobility of spermatozoids.
- Stop smoking.

- Decrease alcohol consumption.
- Decrease coffee consumption.
- Eat healthy and increase the intake of vitamins and minerals, especially zinc.

Do a regular medical checkup to get an early diagnosis and to control diabetes mellitus, as it may predispose a man to erectile problems.

Limit sexual partners, as sexually transmissible diseases may lead to infertility.

Be active and exercise on a regular basis.[xiii]

CAUSES OF INFERTILITY IN FEMALES

1. Failure to ovulate because the hormonal secretion is insufficient or absent because of age or because of some conditions like ovary cancer, radiotherapy, chemotherapy, hormonal treatment, thyroid diseases, hyperprolactinemia, Cushing's disease, malfunction of the hypothalamus, malfunction of the pituitary gland, tumors and surgical ablation of ovaries, diabetes mellitus, kidney diseases, sickle cell anemia, etc.

2. Blockage of fallopian tubes; in most cases, this is a consequence of pelvic inflammatory diseases and STDs.
3. Absence of a uterus
4. Abnormality of the uterus
5. Fibroid uterus
6. Scarred womb as a result of a severe womb infection
7. Cervical incompetence; this happens mostly to women having a history of abortion. (In this specific case, a woman may conceive and end up having a miscarriage.)
8. Endometriosis
9. The presence of spermatozoid antibodies[xiv]

TREATMENT

For both males and females, the treatment depends on the cause of infertility.

CONCLUSION

A couple trying to bear a child must plan for it and consult a gynecologist from the time the decision is made as the process may require patience. This will save you time and help you to avoid stress, as the older you get, the lesser are your chances of conception.

[i] Linda, et al, 2012, "Uterus," MedlinePlus medical encyclopedia, image found at www.nlm.nih.gov/../19263.htm
[ii] "Vagina" found at www.wikipedia.org/wiki/vagina
[iii] Definition of fallopian tube found at www.medterms.com/script/main/ art.as...
Fallopian tube found at www.wikipedia.org/wiki/Fallopiantube
Fallopian tube, *Encyclopaedia Britannica*, found at www.britanica.com

[iv] Ovarian disorders, MedlinePlus, found at www.nlh.nih.gov/MedlinePlus/Ovarian...
[v] Body basics, female reproductive system: about human reproduction, found at www.kidshealth.org>Kids health>Parents>General health

[vi] Follicule ovarian, www.wikipedia.org/wiki/../follicule ovarian Cancer info, En savoir plus sur les hormones feminines, found at www.e.cancer.fr>accueil>info patient>Les cancers>cancer du sein>hormonotherapy

Eureka santé, Les hormones feminines et le cycle menstrual, Que faire en cas d'oublie de la pillule? J'ai oublie ma pillule, www.eurekasante.fr>Accueil>Maladies>Sexualite et contraception
Hypothalamus found at www.wikipedia.org/wiki/hypothalamus
Hypophyse, Futura-sante,www.futura-sciences.com/fr/definition...
Dr Aly Abbara, 2012, "Oestrogenes," www.aly-abbara.com/../oestrogenes.html
Progesterone, www.wikipedia.org/wiki/progest%25C3%...

[vii] Cycle et ovulation, www.doctissimo.fr/htm/sexualite/education
Cancer info, En savoir plus sur les hormones feminines, found at www.e.cancer.fr>accueil>info patient>Les cancers>cancer du sein>hormonotherapy.
Eureka santé, Les hormones feminines et le cycle menstrual, Que faire en cas d'oublie de la pillule? J'ai oublie ma pillule, www.eurekasante.fr>Accueil>Maladies>Sexualite et contraception
Hypothalamus found at www.wikipedia.org/wiki/hypothalamus
Hypophyse, Futura-sante,www.futura-sciences.com/fr/definition...
Dr Aly Abbara, 2012, Oestrogenes, www.aly-abbara.com/../oestrogenes.html
Progesterone, www.wikipedia.org/wiki/progest%25C3%...

[viii] Best fertility monitor, www.bestfertility monitor.com/

[ix] How to get pregnant, boosting fertility found at www.wikihow.com>Home>Categories>Family life>Parenting>Development Stages.
[x] How to get pregnant, boosting fertility found at www.wikihow.com>Home>Categories>Family life>Parenting>Development Stages.
Erin Cleman, RD, LD, "Diet for women who want to become pregnant" found at www.livestrong.com>Home>Family health>Fertility>Fertility Diets
[xi] Infertility diagnostic, found at www.nhs.uk/../fertility-tests.aspx
[xii] Infertility diagnostic, found at www.nhs.uk/../fertility-tests.aspx
[xiii] Getting pregnant found at www.mayoclinic.com>Home>Healthy life style>Getting pregnant>In-Depth

[xiv] Thyroid disease,
www.thyroid.about.com>about.com>Health>Thyroid
disease>Hormone?Fertility/Women
"What affects your fertility?" found at
www.bbc.co.uk/Science/0/21755753
Fertility tests found at www.nhs.uk/../fertility-tests.aspx
First response found at www.firstreponse.com/fertility Tests...